# Mastering Renal Health

**The Comprehensive Health Series**

Paul Sterling

Published by Digital Mind, 2023.

While every precaution has been taken in the preparation of this book, the publisher assumes no responsibility for errors or omissions, or for damages resulting from the use of the information contained herein.

MASTERING RENAL HEALTH

**First edition. December 29, 2023.**



ISBN: 979-8223540281

Written by Paul Sterling.

# Also by Paul Sterling

**Mejora tu Calidad de Vida**
Domina tu Salud Renal

**The Comprehensive Health Series**
Mastering Gastritis: Comprehensive Guide to Understanding and Treating Acute, Chronic, and Erosive Gastritis, plus Stomach Inflammation Management
Managing Diabetes: Understanding and Controlling Type 1, Type 2, and Gestational Diabetes, Practical Strategies for Blood Sugar Management and Lifestyle Adaptation
Mastering Renal Health

# Table of Contents

# Introduction

The kidneys are true silent heroes, working tirelessly to maintain our internal balance. Kidney wellness is an essential part of our overall health, and understanding how to care for these faithful guardians is the key to a journey toward a full, healthy life.

This book seeks to illuminate the path towards understanding and caring for our kidneys in a way that is accessible and understandable to everyone. In a world full of information, often complex and overwhelming , simplicity is our ally. Here, we'll dive into the fascinating world of kidney health, exploring everything from its fundamentals to practical strategies to keep these vital organs in their best shape.

It is essential to understand the vital role that kidneys play in our body. They are not just filters that remove waste, but meticulous architects of internal balances. The kidneys regulate the amount of water in our body, control blood pressure, produce crucial hormones, and filter the blood to remove toxins. In short, they are the guardians of internal harmony, playing a crucial role in keeping us healthy and balanced.

However, despite their importance, kidneys are often neglected until problems arise. The prevalence of kidney diseases is increasing, and many of them are preventable with proper knowledge and kidney care practices. This book is intended to be your trusted guide on the journey toward understanding and caring for your kidneys, helping you make informed decisions to preserve this precious asset of your health.

We'll explore the risk factors that can affect kidney health, from genetics to lifestyle habits, and provide you with tools to evaluate and reduce these risks. It is not just about knowing, but about acting; Therefore, we will present daily habits and lifestyle changes that you can easily incorporate to promote long-term kidney health. From proper hydration to the importance of a balanced diet, we will address each aspect with a practical, action-oriented approach.

Additionally, we will understand the warning signals that our kidneys can send when something is not right. Many times, the initial symptoms can go unnoticed, but learning to recognize these early signs can make the difference in timely detection and treatment. Prevention is key, and awareness of symptoms provides a valuable tool to proactively care for our kidney health.

We will also address common myths and misconceptions about kidney health. Misinformation can be just as damaging as a lack of knowledge, and we'll unravel the misunderstandings to give you a clear and accurate view of what it really means to take care of your kidneys.

Kidneys deserve our diligent attention and care, and this book is designed to guide you, step by step, on the path to healthy kidneys and a fulfilling life. Get ready to embark on this journey that will transform the way you see and care for your kidneys!

# Chapter 1: Understanding Kidney Health

First, think of the kidneys as guardians. Guardians of what? Well, many important things. They control the amount of water in your body, like a captain ensuring that the ship (your body) does not sink or flood. They are also like architects who build internal balances, working hard to make everything work perfectly.

Imagine that your kidneys are magic filters. What do these filters do? They filter the blood to get rid of bad things and keep the good things. It's like when you make a smoothie and use a strainer to remove the seeds and keep only the good stuff. Your kidneys do something like that, but big and all the time.

But here's the thing: sometimes, without you knowing it, your kidneys can be under pressure. They may face challenges that affect their superhero work. And that is what we are going to explore in this chapter. We'll understand what can put your kidneys in trouble and how we can help them remain the brave heroes they are.

## 1.1 Anatomy and Function of the Kidneys

Imagine that your kidneys are like two beans located in the lower part of your back, one on each side of your spine. They are like two hidden treasures that work in the shadows to maintain balance in your body. Each kidney is covered by a type of protective layer called the " renal capsule." This capsule is like armor that protects your kidney heroes from bumps and scratches.

Now, inside those magic beans, there is something incredible: a series of little tubes and filters that do a phenomenal job. These little tubes are called "renal tubules," and they're like little workers that help filter your blood and get rid of things your body doesn't need.

Your kidneys are like a control center. Each kidney has something called the "renal pelvis," which is like a meeting room where all the waste and filtered fluids are collected before being sent out of the body. It's like your kidneys are a cleaning crew, making sure your body gets rid of things that could cause problems.

### Kidney Function: More Than Just Filtering

It is truly incredible the function that these small organs play. In simple terms, kidneys are like the guardians of water quality in your body. They control the amount of water you need and remove the excess to maintain a perfect balance. It's like they have a magic wand to adjust the water level in your body as needed.

But that is not all. Your kidneys are also masters of blood pressure. They regulate pressure by ensuring that the correct amount of fluids and salts are present in your blood. Imagine your kidneys as traffic controllers, keeping everything moving smoothly to avoid congestion and blockages.

Now, here comes the really amazing part: your kidneys are hormone factories. Yes, you heard right. They produce hormones like erythropoietin, which tells your body when it's time to make more red blood cells. They are like little conductors of an orchestra, coordinating all the parts of your body so that they work together in perfect harmony.

### How do they filter blood?

But how does he do all this? It's time to dive a little deeper into the kidney filtration process. Imagine blood as a river flowing throughout your body, carrying good things and some you no longer need. Your kidneys are like the guardians of the river, making sure that only the good continues its path.

First, blood enters the kidneys and passes through those magical little tubes, the renal tubules. Here, kidney workers work hard to separate what is useful from what must go. Everything you don't need, like waste and excess water, heads to the renal pelvis, ready to be expelled.

After this filtration process, the blood returns to its path, now cleaner and ready to continue nourishing your body. It's like your kidneys are the best blood cleaners, making sure everything is in order.

Your kidneys are like low-key superheroes, working tirelessly to keep you in good shape. From filtering blood to regulating blood pressure and producing essential hormones, these small organs play a crucial role in your health.

# 1.2 Risk Factors for Kidney Diseases

**A) What are Risk Factors?**

First, let's clarify what "risk factors" means. They are like warning signs telling us to pay attention and be cautious. In the case of kidney health, these factors are things that could increase your chances of having kidney problems. Imagine them as dark clouds in the sky that could become a storm if we don't take action.

**B) Genetics: DNA and Heredity**

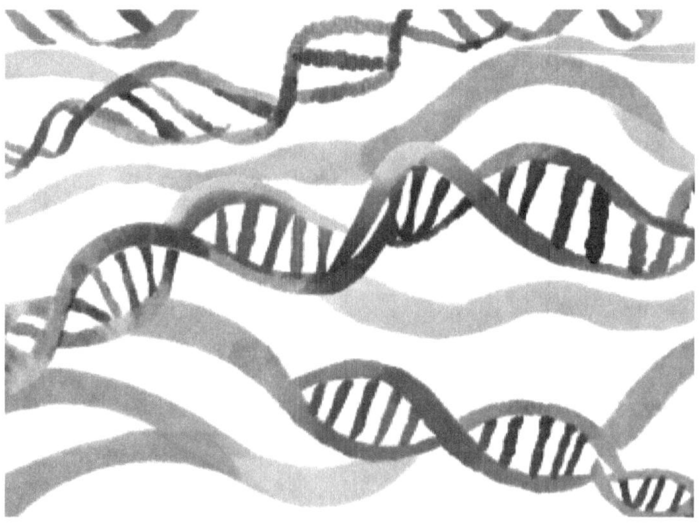

One of the first clouds we could see is genetics, and no, we are not talking about a complicated scientific language. Genetics is about the things we inherit from our parents, like eye color or hair type. In the world of kidneys, some problems can run in the family. If your parents or grandparents had kidney problems, it's like there's a yellow caution light. It doesn't mean you're doomed, but it's a sign that you should be alert and take good care of your kidneys.

**C) High Blood Pressure: A Dangerous Tide**

Another dark cloud that we could see is high blood pressure. What's that? Imagine that your arteries are like the highways that transport blood throughout your body. If these highways become very narrow or have many potholes, blood will have trouble moving. High blood pressure is like when traffic is congested and things are not going as well as they should. This can put a lot of pressure on your kidneys, and over time, could cause damage. Keeping your blood pressure under control is like opening up those highways so everything flows smoothly.

### D) Diabetes: A Dangerous Flame

Now, let's talk about diabetes, another dark cloud that could appear. Diabetes is like a flame that can affect many aspects of your body, including your kidneys. When you have diabetes, your body may have trouble handling sugar, and that can affect your kidneys. It's like a small spark can light a big fire. Keeping diabetes under control is like putting out that spark and protecting your kidneys from possible damage.

### E) Age and Gender: Navigating the Waters of Time

Another important aspect to mention is age and gender. As we age, our bodies change too. Over time, your kidneys may not work as efficiently as they did when you were younger. But, don't worry too much! It is a natural part of life. Additionally, at some stages of life, such as during pregnancy, women may face additional challenges. It's like navigating the waters of time: as you progress, it's important to be aware and take steps to keep your kidneys in good shape.

### F) Lifestyle: Our Boats and How We Sail Them

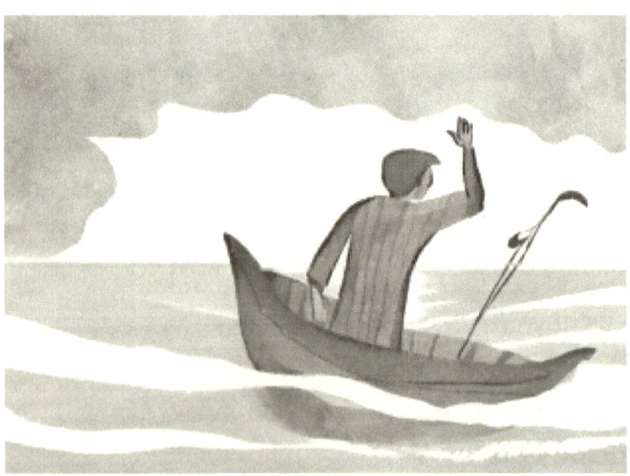

Finally, we come to a crucial point: lifestyle. How do we care for our ships in this vast ocean of life? Here, we talk about everyday habits like what we eat, how much we move, and whether or not we smoke. If we fill our bodies with unhealthy foods or subject them to tobacco smoke, we are creating stormy conditions for our kidneys. But don't worry, changing small things in your lifestyle can be like adjusting the sails on your boat for a smoother ride.

Risk factors are like warning signs on our kidney journey. Genetics, high blood pressure, diabetes, age, gender and our lifestyle are the dark clouds that we could encounter along the way. But here's the good news: we can navigate carefully and avoid storms. Stay aware of these factors and take steps to take care of our kidneys.

# 1.3 Importance of Early Detection

**1. What does "Early Detection" mean?**

Before continuing we must clarify what "early detection" means. It's like when you detect the first drops of rain and decide to carry an umbrella. In the world of kidney health, it means discovering any kidney problems before they become more serious. It's like having a compass that guides you to avoid unnecessary storms on your health.

**2. Silent Signals: Why the Kidneys Speak in Whispers**

The kidneys are fairly silent organs. They don't scream when something is wrong; Rather, they speak in whispers, and sometimes those whispers are difficult to hear. That's why early detection is like paying attention to those whispers before they become a scream. If we can hear those signals early, we can take steps to make sure our kidneys are happy and healthy.

**3. The Magic of Screening Tests: How Do We Know If Everything is OK?**

Now, let's talk about the magic of screening tests. These tests are like the tools doctors use to see what is happening inside our kidneys. Some of these tests can measure the amount of certain substances in the blood or urine, while others can show pictures of the kidneys. It's as if doctors have a magic magnifying glass to closely examine how your kidneys are working.

Getting screened doesn't mean something is definitely wrong. It's like doing a regular checkup on your car to make sure everything is working properly, even if there are no obvious signs of problems. By catching any problems early, we can take action before they become something bigger and more complicated.

**4. Prevention Instead of Cure: The Key to a Healthy Kidney Life**

Early detection is like opening a map and finding a safer route on our kidney journey. It allows us to prevent instead of cure. Why wait for major problems to appear when we can act before they become too complicated? It's like avoiding a storm instead of facing it unprepared.

Imagine that your kidneys are lighthouses in the darkness. Early detection is like making sure those headlights are on and shining bright. They guide us, warn us and help us avoid reefs and dangerous waters.

### 5. Risk Factors: Detect Shadows on the Horizon

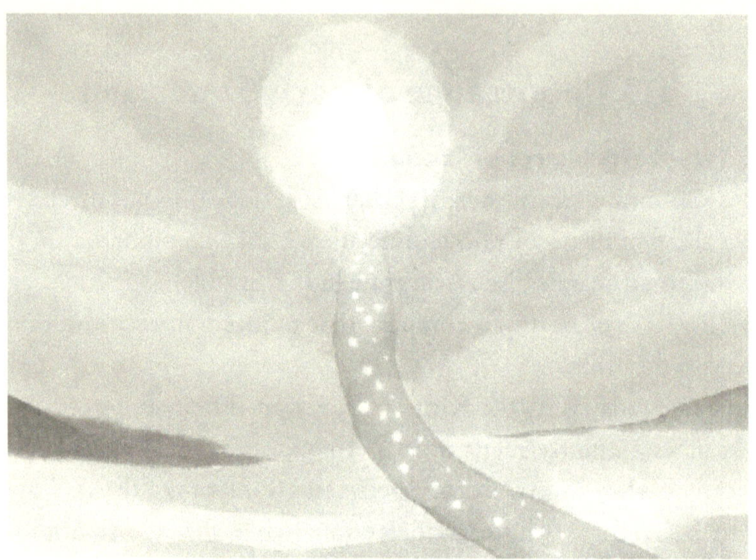

We've talked before about risk factors, those dark clouds on our kidney journey. This is where early detection becomes even more important. If we know our risk factors, we can be even more vigilant. It's as if we are watching the horizon to see if there are shadows that could indicate storms on the way. By being aware of these factors, we can act quickly if we notice something out of the ordinary.

### 6. The Power of Prevention: Small Changes, Big Results

Prevention is like the magic shield that protects us from future problems. Once we know our risk factors and screen for them, we are in a powerful position to make changes. Small changes to our lifestyle, such as eating healthier, staying active and controlling blood pressure, can make a big difference. It's like fixing a small leak in our boat before it turns into a big hole.

Early detection is like turning on the light on the path to healthy kidneys. It helps us hear the whispers in our kidneys before they become screams. With regular screening and an understanding of our risk factors, we are equipped to take control of our kidney health. Prevention and early detection are the tools that allow us to safely navigate the waters of life, avoiding storms and keeping our kidneys healthy.

# Chapter 2: Diabetic Kidney Disease: Breaking Down the Basics

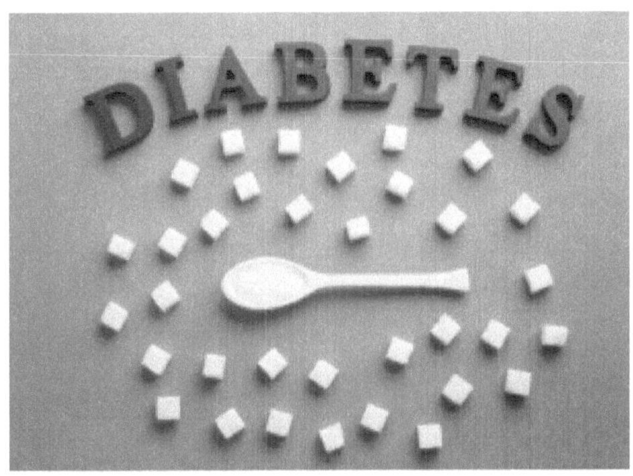

In this chapter we are going to delve into the fundamentals of how diabetes impacts the kidneys. Understanding these fundamentals is like having a map that shows us where obstacles might arise. When we understand how diabetes affects our kidneys, we are better equipped to make informed decisions about how to care for these vital organs.

This chapter is not just about understanding Diabetic Kidney Disease; It's also about learning how to take care of our kidneys despite living with diabetes. We'll explore healthy eating habits, the importance of controlling blood sugar levels, and how to work as a team with our doctors to keep our kidneys in the best shape possible.

## 2.1 Relationship Between Diabetes and Kidney Disease

### 1. What Does the Relationship Between Diabetes and Kidney Disease Mean?

Imagine that diabetes and Diabetic Kidney Disease are like traveling companions in your body. Diabetes is a traveler that sometimes brings with it changes that can affect your kidneys. Diabetic Kidney Disease is like a stop on that journey where we notice how diabetes has left its mark on our kidney heroes.

Diabetes affects the way our body handles sugar, and this alteration can directly influence the health of our kidneys. It's as if diabetes puts our kidneys to the test, and understanding this relationship helps us make informed decisions to protect these vital organs.

## 2. How Diabetes Can Affect Your Kidneys

Let's break down how this connection occurs. Diabetes can cause the blood vessels in the kidneys to narrow and become harder to work. It is as if the highways that carry blood to the kidneys have slower traffic. This narrowing can make it difficult for the kidneys to filter blood properly.

Additionally, diabetes can cause the kidneys to retain more water and salt than normal. This is as if your kidneys are under extra pressure, like when there is too much traffic on a highway. Over time, this extra pressure can cause damage to the kidneys and affect their ability to function properly.

## 3. Importance of Controlling Diabetes to Protect your Kidneys

Now, here comes the crucial part: controlling diabetes is like keeping any storm that could affect your kidneys at bay. If we keep blood sugar levels within a healthy range, we are helping our kidneys to work in optimal conditions.

Imagine diabetes like a juggler in a show. The better the juggler is at balancing the balls, the less likely it is that one will fall and cause problems. In the same way, controlling diabetes is like becoming expert jugglers who keep everything in balance to avoid complications in our kidneys.

## 4. Early Detection: The Light that Guides the Way

We have talked about the importance of early detection in previous chapters, and here it becomes even more relevant. Early detection allows us to identify any changes in our kidneys due to diabetes before they become a bigger problem. It's like turning on headlights in the dark to illuminate any problematic path.

The sooner we discover any signs that something is wrong, the sooner we can take steps to protect our kidneys. Early detection is the key to intervening early and ensuring that our kidneys continue to be the brave heroes of our health.

## 5. Taking Care of Your Kidneys: A Collaborative Journey

The relationship between diabetes and Diabetic Kidney Disease teaches us that taking care of our kidneys is a collaborative journey. Working hand in hand with our doctors, following healthy eating habits and controlling diabetes are powerful actions that allow us to keep our kidneys in excellent shape.

This journey is not just about understanding the relationship between diabetes and Diabetic Kidney Disease; It's about taking measures to protect and strengthen our kidneys on this journey. So, let's continue exploring together and learning how to take care of our kidneys as we continue our exciting journey to healthy kidneys!

## 2.2 Symptoms and Diagnosis of Diabetic Kidney Disease

**A) Symptoms: Signals that your Kidneys Send You**

The kidneys, although silent, have ways of letting us know if something is not quite right. Symptoms can be like little whispers telling us to pay attention. Here are some signs that could indicate kidney problems, especially if you live with diabetes:

- Changes in Urination: Notice if you urinate more or less than usual. The kidneys regulate the amount of water in your body, and any noticeable changes could be a sign.

- Swelling: If you notice swelling in your legs, ankles, or around your eyes, it could be an indicator that your kidneys are not removing excess fluid as they should.

- Fatigue and Weakness: The buildup of waste in the blood due to kidney problems can cause fatigue and weakness. If you feel like you don't have energy as usual, it's important to pay attention.

- Trouble Concentrating: The kidneys also help keep certain chemicals in your body balanced. When they are not working well, you may experience difficulty concentrating.

- Itchy Skin: The buildup of waste in the blood can also cause itchy skin. If you experience this symptom, it is an indication that something may not be right.

It is important to remember that these symptoms are not exclusive to Diabetic Kidney Disease and may be due to other conditions. If you experience any of these symptoms, it is essential to consult your doctor for an accurate diagnosis.

### B) Diagnosis: Deciphering the Language of the Kidneys

When we go to the doctor with concerns about our kidneys, they perform a series of tests to figure out what 's going on. These tests are like specialized tools that help doctors understand the language of our kidneys. Here are some of the common tests that might be performed:

**Blood Tests:** Doctors can test certain substances in the blood, such as creatinine and urea, to evaluate kidney function. High levels of these substances could indicate kidney problems.

**Urine Analysis:** A urine analysis can reveal the presence of proteins or red blood cells, signs of possible kidney problems.

**Glomerular Filtration Rate (GFR):** This test measures how quickly the kidneys filter blood. A low GFR could indicate problems with kidney function.

**Diagnostic Imaging:** In some cases, imaging, such as ultrasound or MRI, may be performed to get a more detailed look at the kidneys and detect possible structural problems.

**Kidney Biopsy:** In more complex situations, a kidney biopsy may be performed to obtain a tissue sample for detailed examination.

These tests are part of the diagnostic process, and each provides valuable information about the health of your kidneys. It's like solving a puzzle, where each piece reveals a different aspect of the situation.

### C) The Importance of Early Detection in Diagnosis

We once again find the importance of early detection in this context. By testing regularly, even if you don't experience obvious symptoms, doctors can detect problems at an early stage. This is crucial because often the symptoms of Diabetic Kidney Disease may not appear until the damage is already done.

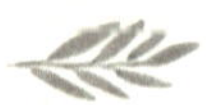

**D) How to Prepare for Medical Consultations**

When you go to the doctor, it helps to be prepared. Carry information about your medical history, including any symptoms you have noticed. If you are taking medications or supplements, have that list handy. Also, don't hesitate to ask questions. Understanding the diagnostic process and the tests performed will give you a greater sense of control over your kidney health.

The symptoms and diagnosis of Diabetic Kidney Disease are like understanding the language our kidneys speak. Paying attention to the signals they send us through symptoms and undergoing regular medical tests are essential steps to keep our kidneys healthy.

# 2.3 Prevention and Control Strategies

## Diabetes Control: The Rudder of the Renal Ship

Diabetes and Diabetic Kidney Disease are intertwined, but there are ways to maintain control. Controlling diabetes is like taking the helm of a ship. When we keep blood sugar levels within a healthy range, we are helping our kidneys work efficiently. This involves following your doctor's orders, taking medications as prescribed, and making lifestyle adjustments, such as eating a balanced diet and staying active.

### Healthy Eating Habits: Nutrition as Fuel

The food we eat is like the fuel that feeds our kidneys. Adopting healthy eating habits is crucial to preventing kidney problems. This includes:

Limit Salt and Sugar: Reducing your consumption of foods high in salt and sugar can help control blood pressure and blood sugar levels, benefiting your kidneys.

Include Fruits and Vegetables: These foods are full of essential nutrients and antioxidants that promote kidney health.

Control Portions: Maintaining a proper balance in portions prevents overloading your kidneys.

### Staying Active: Exercise as a Kidney Ally

Regular exercise is like a loyal ally for your kidneys. It helps control blood pressure, improves circulation and contributes to the control of diabetes. It is not necessary to do intense workouts; Even walking, swimming or practicing yoga can make a difference. Check with your doctor before starting any new exercise program to make sure it is safe for you.

### Controlling Blood Pressure: Maintaining a Serene Sea

High blood pressure can put your kidneys under stress. It's like having turbulent waves in a calm sea. Keeping blood pressure in a healthy range is essential. This involves taking medications as prescribed, adopting a healthy lifestyle, and having regular checkups with your doctor to make sure all is calm in that kidney sea.

### Maintaining a Healthy Weight: Lightening the Kidney Burden

Carrying a healthy weight is like lightening the load that your kidneys must bear. Obesity can increase the risk of kidney disease, so maintaining an appropriate weight is a key prevention strategy. This is achieved through a combination of healthy eating habits and regular physical activity.

### Avoiding Tobacco and Alcohol: Breathing Fresh Air for Your Kidneys

Smoking and excessive alcohol consumption can negatively affect your kidneys. Tobacco restricts blood vessels, reducing blood flow to the kidneys, while excessive alcohol can cause direct damage. Avoiding these habits is like providing fresh air to your kidneys, allowing them to function in optimal conditions.

### Perform Regular Checkups: Sailing with the Wind in Your Favor

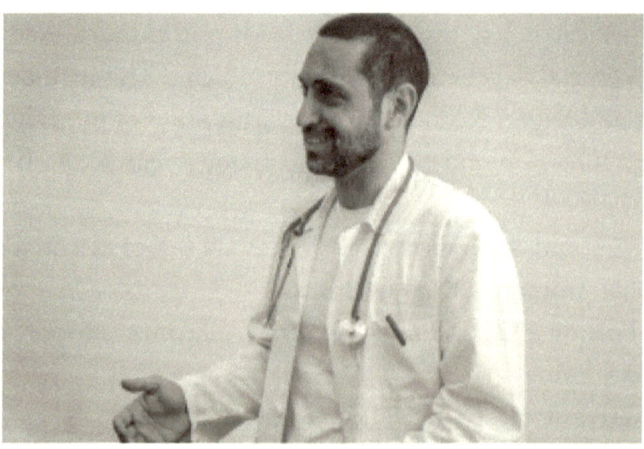

Regular checkups with your doctor are like having the wind at your back on this kidney journey. These checkups include screening tests to evaluate the health of your kidneys and detect any problems early. Be sure to follow your doctor's recommendations and report any changes in your kidney health.

Prevention and control strategies are the tools that will guide your kidneys towards health. Managing diabetes, adopting healthy eating habits, staying active, and taking care of your blood pressure are essential steps. By incorporating these strategies into your daily life, you will be taking firm steps toward healthy kidneys.

# Chapter 3: Chronic Kidney Failure: A Silent Challenge

This chapter is like opening a door to a room where we will explore the challenges our kidneys face when chronic kidney failure occurs. But don't worry, we will be here to understand what it means and how we can deal with it positively. So, get ready to discover more about this challenge and how we can overcome it together on our journey to stronger, healthier kidneys!

## 3.1 Causes and Progression of Chronic Kidney Failure

**A) Causes of Chronic Kidney Failure: Detecting the Roots of the Problem**

Chronic Kidney Failure does not usually appear overnight; It has its roots in various causes. It's like a puzzle where various pieces come together to form the whole picture. Here are some of the most common causes:

- Diabetes: Diabetes can be a major trigger. High blood sugar levels can damage the blood vessels in the kidneys, affecting their ability to filter blood properly.
- High Blood Pressure: High blood pressure can put an extra burden on the kidneys. Over time, this can cause gradual damage to these vital organs.
- Heart Diseases: Heart problems can affect blood circulation, directly impacting kidney health.
- Hereditary Diseases: Some genetic conditions can increase the risk of developing CKD.
- Chronic Infections: Persistent kidney infections can contribute to kidney deterioration.
- Urinary Obstruction: Problems that block the normal flow of urine can

cause damage over time.

- Excessive Medication Consumption: Some medications, if consumed in excess or for long periods, can negatively affect the kidneys.

It is important to remember that these are not the only causes and that CKD can result from a combination of several factors. The key is to recognize and address these causes to prevent or delay disease progression.

**B) Progression of Chronic Kidney Failure: The Silent Journey**

Chronic Kidney Failure is a silent journey that the kidneys take toward a reduced ability to perform their functions. It is like a river that flows slowly, carrying with it the challenges that affect these organs. Let's see how this journey progresses:

1. Initial Phase: At this stage, the kidneys can still perform their basic functions, but may show signs of damage. There may be no obvious symptoms in this phase, making it even more challenging to detect without specific testing.

1. Intermediate Phase: As it progresses, the kidneys' ability to filter blood and remove waste may decrease. Symptoms such as fatigue, bloating, and changes in urination may begin to appear.

1. Advanced Phase: In this stage, kidney function is significantly reduced. Symptoms may intensify, and treatments such as dialysis may be necessary to help the kidneys perform their functions.

1. Terminal Stage: In this last stage, kidney function is highly compromised. A kidney transplant or more intensive treatments may be required to sustain the patient.

**C) Importance of Early Detection: A Light on the Path**

Early detection is like turning on a light on the path of Chronic Kidney Failure. Since symptoms may not be evident in the early stages, regular testing is essential, especially if risk factors such as diabetes or high blood pressure exist. Early detection gives us the opportunity to intervene before the disease progresses significantly.

**D) How to Protect your Kidneys and Reduce the Risk of CRF**

Although CKD can be challenging, there are steps we can take to protect our kidneys and reduce the risk of this condition:

1. Control Diabetes and Blood Pressure: Keeping these two aspects under control is essential.

1. Adopt a Healthy Lifestyle: Habits such as a balanced diet, regular exercise, and avoiding excessive alcohol and tobacco consumption contribute to kidney health.

1. Perform Regular Checkups: Regular screening tests, especially if there are risk factors, are essential.

1. Consult a Health Professional: If you experience symptoms such as changes in urination, swelling or fatigue, do not hesitate to consult a doctor.

Understanding the causes and progression of Chronic Kidney Failure is essential to addressing this silent challenge. By recognizing early signs and taking preventive measures, we can significantly contribute to the health of our kidneys.

# 3.2 Available Treatments: Dialysis and Kidney Transplant

## Dialysis: Filtering Life

When the kidneys can't do their job of filtering waste and fluid effectively, dialysis comes into the picture as a temporary hero. Dialysis is a treatment that helps perform functions that the kidneys can no longer perform. Imagine dialysis as an additional filter that helps purify your blood. There are two main types of dialysis: hemodialysis and peritoneal dialysis.

- Hemodialysis: This type of dialysis is performed in a specialized center. Blood is removed from your body, filtered through a machine to remove waste, and then returned to your body.

- Peritoneal Dialysis: In this case, a special liquid is introduced into the abdomen through a thin tube. This liquid absorbs waste and then drains away, taking unwanted substances with it.

Dialysis is like a bridge that you can cross while you work to strengthen your kidneys or wait for the possibility of a transplant.

### Kidney Transplant: A New Beginning

Kidney transplant is like a new opportunity for your kidneys. In this treatment, a healthy kidney from a donor is placed in your body, taking the place of your damaged kidneys. It's like changing a part on your body machine to make it work more efficiently.

However, transplants are not always an immediate option, as there is a shortage of donor organs. People on the waiting list can wait months or even years to receive a transplant. In the meantime, dialysis can be a vital solution to maintaining health until the time is right for transplant.

### How to Face These Treatments: Practical Tips

Commitment to Treatment: Both dialysis and transplant require constant commitment. It is important to follow the instructions of the medical team and comply with the scheduled treatments.

1. **Emotional Support:** Facing treatments such as dialysis and transplant can be emotionally challenging. Seeking emotional support, whether from friends, family, or support groups, can make all the difference.

1. **Healthy Lifestyle:** Maintaining a healthy lifestyle is essential during these treatments. This includes following a balanced diet, engaging in physical activity as recommended by your medical team, and avoiding harmful habits such as smoking and excessive alcohol consumption.

1. **Open Communication with the Medical Team:** Maintaining open lines of communication with the medical team is essential. Reporting

any symptoms or concerns can help them adjust treatment as needed.

### The Role of Prevention and Early Detection

Although dialysis and kidney transplant are crucial paths when Chronic Kidney Failure manifests itself, prevention and early detection are always the best tools. Controlling diabetes and blood pressure, adopting healthy lifestyle habits, and having regular checkups are steps that can help avoid reaching the need for these advanced treatments.

Dialysis and kidney transplant are like two important tools in our resource box to face Chronic Kidney Failure. These treatments allow people to move forward, strengthening their kidneys and giving them a new chance at life.

# 3.3 Coping with the Emotional and Social Aspects of Kidney Failure

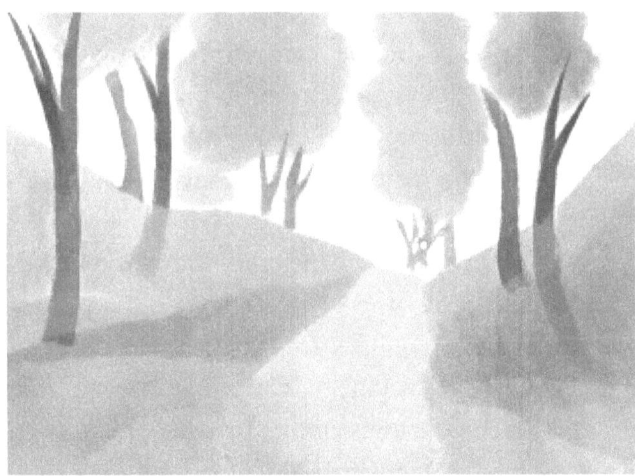

### A) Emotions that May Arise with Chronic Kidney Failure

Facing CKD can be a rollercoaster of emotions. It's completely normal to feel overwhelmed, anxious, or even sad. Here are some common emotions that can arise and how to address them:

Fear and Uncertainty: CKD can bring with it fears about the future and uncertainty about how it will affect your life. It is essential to recognize these feelings and share them with your medical team, friends or family.

Sadness and Loss: Adjusting to the reality of CKD can lead to feelings of sadness and loss. You may feel like you are losing part of your old life. Talking about these feelings with loved ones or a health professional can help ease the emotional burden.

Stress and Anxiety: Managing treatments, lifestyle changes, and health concerns can cause stress and anxiety. Establishing habits to manage stress, such as meditation or light exercise, can be beneficial.

Impact on Self-Esteem: CKD can affect self-image and self-esteem. Recognizing and celebrating achievements, even small ones, can help maintain a positive self-image.

**B) The Importance of Support Networks**

When you face CKD, you are not alone. Building and maintaining support networks is essential. Here are some ways to weave these webs:

- Open Communication: Talking openly with friends, family or health professionals about your emotions is an important step. Open communication builds bridges that connect you with those around you.
- Support Groups: Joining support groups, whether in person or online, allows you to connect with people who are going through similar experiences. Sharing experiences and advice can be comforting and helpful.
- Family Participation: Involving the family in your process can strengthen emotional support. Sharing information about CRI and how they can help can build a strong base of support.
- Mental Health Professionals: Consulting with a mental health professional, such as a counselor or psychologist, can provide tools to manage the emotional impact of CKD.

**C) Adapting to Social and Labor Changes**

CRI can influence your social and work life. Here are some tips to adapt to these changes:

Communication at Work: Talking to your employer about your situation and exploring options such as flexible hours or adjustments to assignments can help keep you active in the workplace.

Adjusted Social Life: Adapting your social life to your needs can include doing less strenuous activities or planning outings at times of the day when you feel better.

Explore New Opportunities: If changes in health impact your career, exploring new opportunities or skills can open unexpected avenues.

Establish Limits: Recognizing your limits is key. Don't be afraid to say no when necessary and prioritize your well-being.

**D) Personal Care and Mental Health**

Taking care of yourself is an essential component when facing CKD. Here are some useful practices:

**Adequate Rest:** Getting enough sleep is essential for recovery and mainly for stress management.

**Adjusted Physical Activity:** Staying active within your limits can improve mood and overall health.

**Healthy Eating:** A balanced diet contributes not only to your kidneys but also to your general well-being.

Find Moments of Joy: Even in the midst of challenges, finding moments of joy and gratitude can strengthen a positive mindset.

Facing the emotional and social aspects of Chronic Kidney Failure is like weaving a strong and resilient support network . Through open communication, family involvement, seeking professional support, and self-care, you can bravely confront these issues.

# Chapter 4: Dialysis: Navigating the Waters of Renal Therapy

In this chapter of our journey to kidney health, we will dive into the waters of dialysis, a vital therapy for those facing challenges in the functioning of their kidneys. Dialysis is like a bridge that helps filter the blood and remove waste when the kidneys encounter difficulties. We are going to explore two important routes in this journey: hemodialysis and renal peritoneal dialysis. Imagine these options as paths that adapt to different needs and circumstances, each with its own characteristics. We're here to break down these options in a clear and accessible way, so you can understand how these therapies can strengthen your kidneys in your quest for kidney health.

## 4.1 Types of Dialysis: Hemodialysis and Peritoneal Dialysis

### Hemodialysis: The Path of Extracorporeal Filtration

Hemodialysis is like a scheduled trip to a specialized station to filter your blood. Here are some keys to understand this route:

1. The Hemodialysis Center: Hemodialysis is usually performed in a specialized center. Imagine this place as a service station for your kidneys, where a trained team is in charge of carrying out the filtering process.

2. The Hemodialysis Machine: During hemodialysis, your blood is removed from your body and directed to a specialized machine. This machine acts as a filter that removes waste and excess fluid from the blood.

3. Duration and Frequency: Hemodialysis sessions usually last several hours and are performed several times a week, depending on the needs of each individual. It is a regular commitment, but vital to maintain kidney health.

### Advantages of Hemodialysis

1. Filtering Efficiency: Hemodialysis is effective in removing waste and fluid from the blood quickly.

2. Professional Supervision: As it is carried out in a specialized center, it has the constant supervision of health professionals.

3. Renal Peritoneal Dialysis: An Autonomous Journey in Your Own Space

Now, let's switch gears and explore renal peritoneal dialysis, an option that gives you more autonomy in your blood filtration journey. Here are some keys to understand this route:

**1. At Home:** Peritoneal dialysis can be performed in the comfort of your home. Imagine your family space as the center of operations for this therapy.

**2. The Peritoneum as a Natural Filter:** Instead of an external machine, peritoneal dialysis uses the peritoneum, a membrane in your abdomen, as a natural filter. A special fluid is introduced into the abdomen and absorbs waste and excess fluid. This fluid is then drained, taking unwanted substances with it.

**3. Multiple Cycles:** Renal peritoneal dialysis involves several cycles throughout the day and night. This more distributed approach provides a continuous form of filtering.

<u>**Advantages of Renal Peritoneal Dialysis**</u>

Greater Autonomy: When performed at home, it provides greater autonomy and flexibility compared to hemodialysis.

Fewer Dietary Restrictions: Some people find that peritoneal dialysis allows for a less restrictive diet compared to hemodialysis.

Both dialysis options are like routes that can lead us to our destination of healthier kidneys. The choice between hemodialysis and renal peritoneal dialysis is often based on factors such as personal preferences, lifestyle, and individual medical needs. It's like having options on a trip, where you choose the route that best suits you.

<u>**How to Choose the Right Route for You**</u>

a. Lifestyle: Consider your daily routine, your commitments and your treatment preferences. Do you value autonomy and flexibility at home, or do you prefer professional supervision in a center?

a. General Health: Individual medical conditions can influence the choice of dialysis. Your medical team will guide you in the right direction based on your specific health needs.

a. Support and Education: Getting information and educational support about both options will help you make informed decisions. Talk to your medical team and participate in dialysis educational programs.

a. Adaptability to Changes: Consider how each option adapts to possible changes in your life. Adaptability is key to maintaining consistency in your treatment.

Hemodialysis and renal peritoneal dialysis are like two paths that lead to kidney health. Both offer effective ways to filter the blood and keep the kidneys functioning. By understanding the features and advantages of each route, you will be better equipped to make informed decisions on your kidney journey.

# 4.2 Dialysis Process: What to Expect and How to Prepare

**1. Preparations for the Dialysis Session**

Before starting dialysis, there are some key preparations:

Vascular Access: If you are opting for hemodialysis, vascular access, such as a catheter or fistula, will be needed. This access provides a route for blood to flow to and from the dialysis machine.

Positioning on the Machine: In the case of hemodialysis, you will be connected to the machine through your vascular access. For peritoneal dialysis, the process is usually done at home, and your medical team will provide you with the necessary equipment.

**2. During the Dialysis Session**

The dialysis process involves several stages as the blood is filtered to remove waste and extra fluid. Some key aspects include:

1. Blood Filtering: In hemodialysis, blood is removed from the body and directed to the dialysis machine, where it is filtered before returning to the body. In peritoneal dialysis, special fluid is introduced into the abdomen and absorbs waste before being drained.

2. Constant Monitoring: During the dialysis session, your medical team will constantly monitor the process. In hemodialysis, this occurs in a specialized center, while peritoneal dialysis allows greater autonomy at home.

3. Session Duration: The duration of each session may vary. Hemodialysis usually takes several hours and is performed several times a week. Peritoneal dialysis involves cycles spread throughout the day and night.

**3. After the Dialysis Session**

After completing your dialysis session, it is important to keep a few key things in mind:

1. Recovery: A short recovery time may be necessary, especially after hemodialysis. You may feel tired, but this feeling usually decreases over time.

2. Hydration and Nutrition: After dialysis, staying hydrated and following a balanced diet is essential. Your medical team can offer specific guidelines.

3. Medical Follow-up: Maintaining regular medical follow-up is essential. Your medical team will review your progress and make adjustments as necessary.

**4. How to Prepare Mentally and Emotionally**

Preparation for dialysis is not just limited to the physical; Mental and emotional health are also crucial. Here are some tips:

- Continuing Education: Getting detailed information about the dialysis process helps you feel more prepared and empowered.
- Open Communication: Talk to your medical team about any concerns or questions you may have. Open communication strengthens trust and mutual understanding.
- Emotional Support: Seeking support from friends, family, or support groups can be comforting. Sharing your feelings and experiences can ease the emotional burden.
- Establish Routines: Establishing daily routines that include time for self-care and enjoyable activities can help maintain a positive mindset.

**5. Important Aspects to Consider**

Space Conditions at Home: If you are opting for peritoneal dialysis at home, make sure you have a clean and organized space to carry out the process.

Rigorous Hygiene: Hygiene is essential to prevent infections, especially in the case of peritoneal dialysis where the special liquid is handled.

Time Planning: Adjusting your schedule to accommodate dialysis sessions and recovery times is essential. Proper planning makes it easier to integrate dialysis into your daily life.

The dialysis process is like sailing in specific waters to maintain kidney health. Understanding what to expect, how to prepare, and taking care of your emotional well-being are key components of this journey. By looking at this process as a tool to strengthen your kidneys, you can approach it with confidence and determination. Let's continue exploring together, learning more about the dialysis journey and moving toward strong, healthy kidneys. Onwards on our kidney journey!

# 4.3 Living a Full Life During Dialysis

## A) Maintaining Social Connections

Dialysis does not mean being alone. Maintaining social connections is essential for a fulfilling life. Here are some ways to strengthen your ties:

Participate in Support Groups: Joining support groups allows you to share experiences with people who understand your journey. Connecting with others who are going through similar situations can be comforting.

Involve the Family: Dialysis is not only an individual journey, but also a family one. Involving family in your process creates a strong support system.

Explore Social Activities: Participating in social activities, even virtually, helps you stay connected with friends and loved ones.

## B) Facing Emotional Challenges

Dialysis can trigger a range of emotions, but facing these emotional challenges is an integral part of living fully:

**Talk about your feelings:** Communicating openly and honestly about your feelings with friends, family, or health professionals can ease the emotional burden.

**Seek Professional Support:** Consulting with a mental health professional can give you tools to manage stress and difficult emotions.

**Find Moments of Joy:** Despite the challenges, look for moments of joy in your day. It could be enjoying a special meal, reading a book you are passionate about, or doing an activity you love.

**C) Integrating Healthy Habits**

Maintaining healthy habits is essential for a full life during dialysis:

- Balanced Diet: A balanced diet, adapted to the needs of your treatment, contributes to your general well-being.

- Adjusted Physical Activity: Performing physical activity as directed by your medical team can improve your mood and physical health.

- Personal Care: Self-care, which includes adequate rest and moments of relaxation, is essential for your well-being.

**D) Discovering New Passions**

Dialysis does not limit your ability to discover new passions or enjoy existing activities:

Learn Something New: Explore new skills or interests that you can develop during dialysis sessions or in your free time.

Cultivate Existing Passions: Continue to enjoy the activities you love. Whether it's music, art, or gardening, maintaining these passions enriches your daily life.

Set Small Goals: Setting achievable goals gives you a sense of achievement and motivation. Celebrate every small step on your journey.

**E) Time Planning for Dialysis**

Dialysis is part of your routine, but it is also important to balance your treatment time with other activities:

1. Schedule Breaks: If dialysis sessions are long, schedule breaks to read, listen to music, or enjoy a short walk.

2. Take Advantage of Home Sessions: If you are on peritoneal dialysis at home, you can do some activities while carrying out the process. Listening to a podcast, watching a movie, or reading are options that can make time go by faster.

3. Planning Activities After Dialysis: Organizing enjoyable activities after dialysis sessions gives you something pleasant to look forward to.

Living a full life during dialysis is like discovering strength in each day of your kidney journey. Maintaining social connections, facing emotional challenges, integrating healthy habits, discovering new passions, and planning your time are key strategies. Each day presents opportunities to find meaning, joy, and connection.

# Chapter 5: Kidney Diet: Nutrition for Kidney Wellness

I n this chapter let's explore how our eating habits can play a crucial role in the well-being of our kidneys. Here we will guide you through nutritional options to strengthen your kidneys and improve your overall health. We're here to break down in a simple and accessible way how you can eat for kidney wellness, giving you the tools you need to make informed decisions on your journey to stronger, healthier kidneys. Understanding how to nourish your kidneys wisely through diet is essential for kidney well-being.

## 5.1 Principles of a Healthy Kidney Diet

### 1. Control of Protein Intake

Proteins are like the essential bricks to build and repair our body. However, in the case of compromised kidneys, it is crucial to control the amount of protein we consume. Here are some keys:

Quality over Quantity: Opt for high-quality proteins, such as those found in lean meats, fish, eggs, and low-fat dairy products. These proteins are easier for your kidneys to process.

Portion Monitoring: Controlling protein portions is essential. A nutritionist can help you establish specific guidelines based on your individual needs.

### 2. Management of Sodium Intake

Sodium, found in salt and many processed foods, can affect blood pressure and fluid retention. Here are some strategies to manage sodium intake:

- Cooking with Spices and Herbs: Instead of relying too much on salt, explore the world of spices and herbs to season your meals.

- Read Nutrition Labels: Get familiar with reading labels to identify low-sodium foods. Opt for fresh options and avoid foods high in sodium.

- Avoid Processed Foods: Processed foods often contain high levels of sodium. Opt for fresh foods and prepare your meals whenever possible.

### 3. Control of Phosphorus Intake

Phosphorus, present in foods such as dairy, nuts and certain grains, can accumulate in the body when the kidneys cannot eliminate it efficiently. Here are some suggestions:

Limit Foods Rich in Phosphorus: Control the intake of foods rich in phosphorus, such as strong cheeses, nuts and wheat germ.

Choosing Low-Phosphorus Dairy: Opt for low-phosphorus dairy options, such as skim milk or yogurt.

Food Preparation: Some preparation methods, such as soaking certain grains and legumes, can reduce their phosphorus content.

### 4. Moderate Potassium Consumption

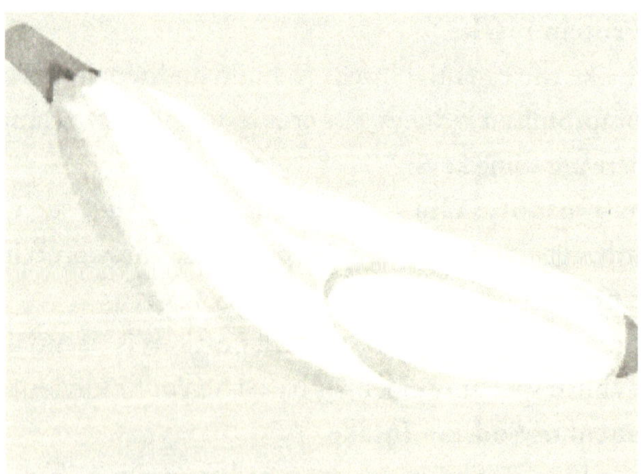

Potassium is essential for health, but its control is crucial when it comes to compromised kidneys. Here are some recommendations:

a) Moderate Fruits and Vegetables: Include fruits and vegetables in your diet, but in moderate quantities. Opt for low potassium options, such as apples, grapes and carrots.

b) Food Processing: Some processing methods, such as boiling certain vegetables, can reduce their potassium content.

c) Balance with Calcium: Maintain an adequate balance between potassium and calcium consumption, since these minerals interact in the body.

## 5. Conscious Hydration

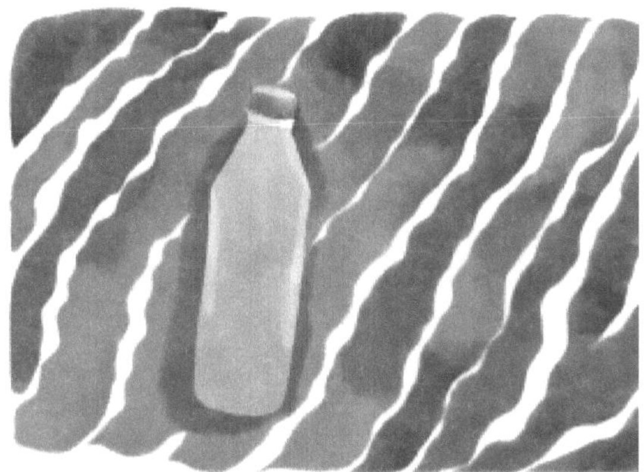

Staying hydrated is key to kidney health, but the amount of fluids can vary depending on individual needs. Here are some suggestions:

1. Listen to your Body: Pay attention to your body's signals. Drink when you are thirsty and adjust your fluid intake as directed by your medical team.

1. Limiting Sugary Drinks: Limit consumption of sugary drinks, as they can contribute to excessive calorie intake and affect overall health.

1. Including Water in Meals: Drinking water during meals can help with digestion and prevent dehydration.

The principles of a healthy kidney diet are like the key tools in your kidney wellness box. Controlling protein intake, managing sodium, controlling phosphorus, moderating potassium, and maintaining conscious hydration are essential steps. Remember that customization is key, and working closely with your medical team and a nutritionist can help you adapt these principles to your specific needs.

## 5.2 Foods to Avoid and Recommended Foods

### Foods to Avoid

- Foods High in Sodium:
    - Avoid Excess Salt: Reduce your intake of processed foods, fast foods and condiments rich in salt. Choose to cook at home and season your meals with herbs and spices.

- Foods Rich in Phosphorus:
    - Control Nuts and Seeds Consumption: Although they are nutritious, limit nuts and seeds, as they can be high in phosphorus. Opt for small portions.

- Foods High in Potassium:
    - Moderate Fruits and Vegetables: Control the consumption of fruits and vegetables high in potassium, such as bananas, oranges and spinach. Choose lower potassium options, such as apples, grapes and carrots.

- Foods with Low Quality Proteins:
    - Limit Processed Meats: Avoid processed meats and sausages, as they may contain low quality protein and additional sodium. Opt for lean proteins such as chicken, fish and eggs.

- Sugary drinks:
    - Reduce Consumption of Sugary Drinks: Limit sugary drinks, as they can contribute to excessive calorie intake and do not provide significant nutritional benefits.

### Recommended Foods

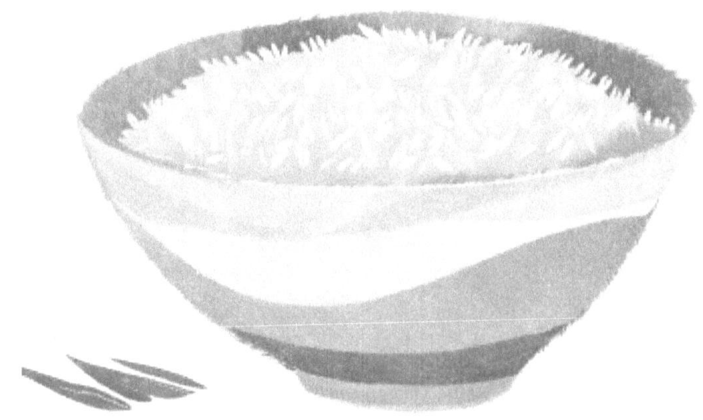

- Green Leafy Vegetables:
    - Spinach, Lettuce, Kale: These vegetables are low in potassium and phosphorus, making them excellent options for a kidney diet.

- Low Potassium Fruits:
    - Apples, Grapes, Pears: These fruits are delicious and provide nutrients without being too high in potassium.

- Cold Water Fish:
    - Salmon, Trout, Tuna: Cold water fish is an excellent source of high-quality protein and omega-3 fatty acids.

- Eggs:
    - Source of Quality Protein: Eggs are rich in high-quality proteins and are versatile in the kitchen.

- Rice and pasta:
    - Low Phosphorus Options: Rice and pasta are low phosphorus starch options and can be part of balanced meals.

- White Bread and Refined Cereals:
  - Low-Phosphorus Alternatives: Opt for white bread and refined grains instead of whole-grain options to limit phosphorus intake.

- Apples and Blueberries:
  - Healthy Fruits: Apples and blueberries are examples of fruits low in potassium and phosphorus, ideal for a kidney diet.

- Olive oil:
  - Healthy Fat: Olive oil is an excellent source of healthy fats and can be used in dressings and cooking.

## **Practical Tips for Daily Nutrition**

- Meal Planning:
  - Prepare Meals at Home: Cooking at home allows you to have control over the ingredients and reduces the intake of processed foods.

- Portion Control:
  - Monitor Amounts: Keep an eye on portion sizes to control nutrient intake.

- Conscious Hydration:
  - Drink Water Regularly: Maintain a healthy fluid balance by drinking water regularly throughout the day.

- Nutritional Counseling:
  - Consult with a Nutritionist: A nutritionist can offer personalized guidance based on your specific needs.

- Food Registry:
  - Keep a Food Log: Keep a record of your food choices to identify patterns and make adjustments as necessary.

Choosing foods wisely in your kidney diet is like navigating the waters to strengthen your kidneys. Avoiding harmful foods and choosing nutritious options will guide you toward optimal kidney well-being. Remember that customization is key, and working collaboratively with your medical team and a nutritionist will allow you to tailor these recommendations to your specific needs.

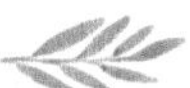

# 5.3 Nutritious and Delicious Recipes for Kidney Patients

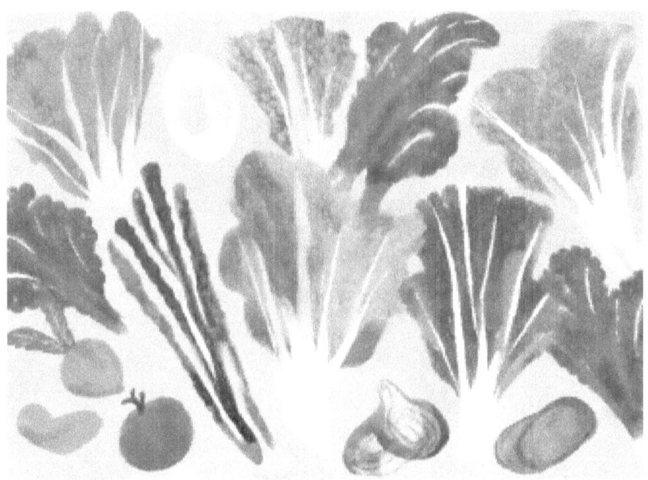

**A) Fresh Quinoa Salad with Vegetables**

Ingredients:

- 1 cup cooked quinoa
- 1 cucumber, cut into cubes
- 1 tomato, chopped
- 1 avocado, sliced
- 1/4 cup black olives, chopped
- 1/4 cup crumbled feta cheese
- 2 tablespoons olive oil

- Juice of 1 lemon
- Salt and pepper to taste

Instructions:

- Mix the cooked quinoa with the vegetables in a large bowl.
- Add the olives and feta cheese.
- In a small bowl, whisk together the olive oil, lemon juice, salt, and pepper to make the dressing.
- Pour the dressing over the salad and toss gently.
- Serve the salad fresh and enjoy this nutrient-packed dish.

## B) Grilled Chicken with Aromatic Herbs

Ingredients:

- 2 boneless, skinless chicken breasts
- 2 tablespoons olive oil
- 1 teaspoon fresh rosemary, chopped
- 1 teaspoon fresh thyme, chopped
- 1 clove garlic, minced
- Salt and pepper to taste

Instructions:

- In a small bowl, whisk together the olive oil, rosemary, thyme and garlic.
- Season the chicken breasts with salt and pepper to taste.
- Spread the herb mixture over the chicken.
- Preheat the grill and cook the chicken until cooked through.
- Serve the grilled chicken with a side of your choice and enjoy this tasty protein option.

## C) Fruit and Spinach Smoothie

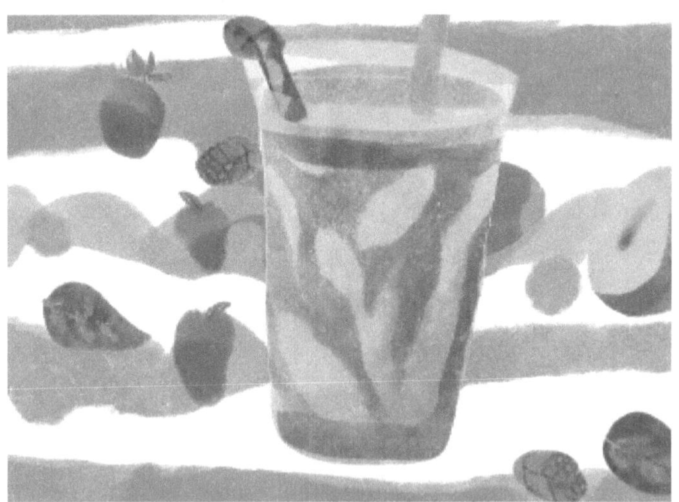

Ingredients:

- 1 ripe banana
- 1 cup fresh pineapple, chopped
- 1 cup fresh spinach
- 1/2 cup nonfat Greek yogurt
- 1 cup of water or lactose-free milk
- Ice to taste

Instructions:

- Place all the ingredients in a blender.
- Blend until smooth.
- Add more liquid if necessary and adjust the amount of ice according to your preference.
- Serve this refreshing and nutrient-packed smoothie.

## D) Lentil Soup with Vegetables

Ingredients:

- 1 cup dried lentils, rinsed
- 1 carrot, cut into cubes

- 1 celery, cut into pieces
- 1 chopped onion
- 2 cloves garlic, minced
- 4 cups low sodium vegetable broth
- 1 bay leaf
- 1 teaspoon ground cumin
- Salt and pepper to taste

Instructions:

- In a large pot, sauté onion and garlic until golden.
- Add the lentils, carrot, celery, vegetable broth, bay leaf and cumin.
- Bring the mixture to a boil and then reduce the heat and simmer until the lentils are tender.
- Season with salt and pepper to taste.
- Serve this comforting soup full of plant proteins.

**E) Grilled Zucchini Garnish**

Ingredients:

- 2 zucchini, sliced
- 2 tablespoons olive oil
- 1 teaspoon dried oregano
- 1 teaspoon dried basil
- Salt and pepper to taste

Instructions:

- Toss the zucchini slices with olive oil, oregano and basil.
- Grill zucchini on a hot grill until tender with grill marks.
- Season with salt and pepper to taste.
- Serve these grilled zucchini as a healthy and delicious side dish.

# Chapter 6: Lifestyle Management: Promoting Kidney Health Every Day

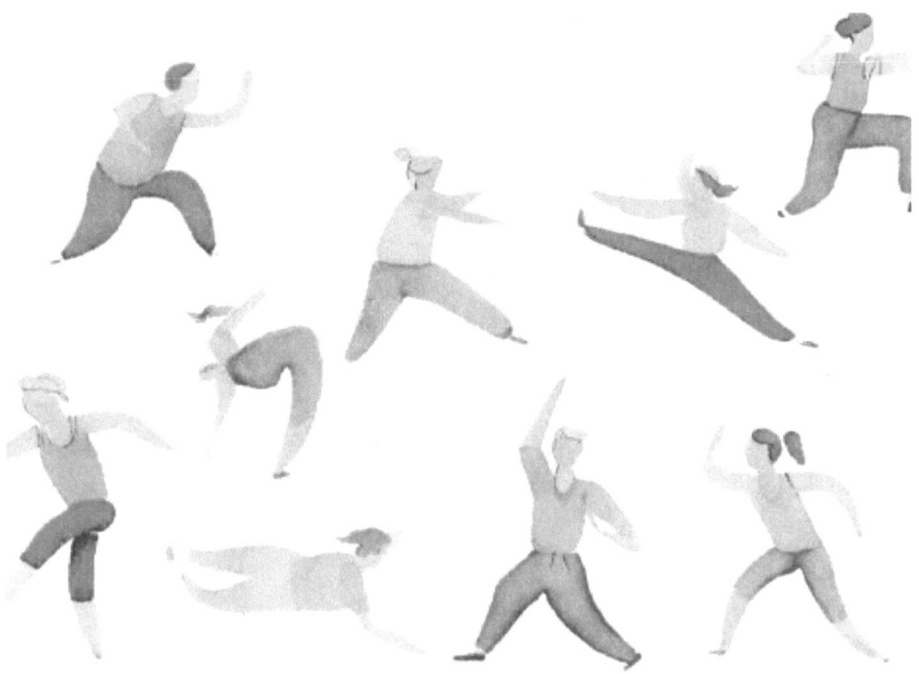

In this leg of our journey towards stronger, healthier kidneys, we will focus on the importance of physical exercise and how it can be a crucial ally for kidney health. Imagine exercise as a traveling companion, walking with you toward optimal kidney wellness. We'll explore clearly and simply why movement is so beneficial and how you can easily incorporate it into your daily routine.

## 6.1 Importance of Physical Exercise in Kidney Health

### 1. Stimulates Blood Circulation

When you exercise, your heart pumps more blood, improving circulation throughout your body, including your kidneys. Blood carries oxygen and essential nutrients to these organs, contributing to their health and optimal functioning.

## 2. Control Blood Pressure

Regular exercise is a powerful tool for controlling blood pressure. Maintaining blood pressure within healthy levels is essential to protect your kidneys, since high blood pressure can damage the blood vessels in these organs.

## 3. Contributes to a Healthy Weight

Maintaining a healthy body weight is beneficial for kidney health. Exercise helps burn calories and maintain a proper balance between energy intake and expenditure. A healthy weight reduces the load on the kidneys and lowers the risk of kidney disease.

## 4. Improves Stamina and Energy

Regular exercise improves endurance and cardiovascular fitness, meaning you'll feel more energetic in your daily life. This can motivate you to maintain healthy habits, such as a balanced diet and proper hydration, which are essential for kidney health.

## 5. Control Blood Sugar Levels

Exercise also plays a crucial role in controlling blood sugar levels. Keeping glucose at healthy levels is essential to prevent kidney problems related to diabetes, a leading cause of chronic kidney disease.

## 6. Promotes Detoxification Through Sweat

The sweat generated during exercise acts as a detoxification pathway for the body. Through perspiration, toxins and waste are eliminated, easing the burden on the kidneys and promoting a cleaner, healthier environment in the body.

## 7. Fight Stress

Stress can have a negative impact on kidney health. Exercise is a great way to combat stress, as it releases endorphins, the so-called "happy hormones", which not only improve your mood but also reduce the emotional burden that stress can put on your kidneys.

## 8. Practical Tips for Incorporating Exercise

- Find an Activity You Enjoy: Choose a physical activity you enjoy to make it part of your routine. It can be walking, swimming, cycling or any activity that you enjoy.

- Start Slowly: If you are new to exercise, start with short sessions and gradually increase the duration and intensity. This helps prevent injuries and build a solid foundation.
- Incorporate Exercise into your Daily Routine: Find ways to incorporate exercise into your daily life. You can choose to climb stairs instead of taking the elevator, walk instead of driving short distances, or stretch while watching TV.

- Check with Your Doctor: Before starting a new exercise program, especially if you have pre-existing medical conditions, check with your doctor to make sure it is safe for you.
- Enjoy Social Activities: Participate in physical activities that you can enjoy with friends or family. Not only does this make exercise more fun, it also strengthens social connections, another key aspect of kidney health.

# 6.2 Stress Control and its Impact on Kidney Function

In this section of our journey to stronger, healthier kidneys, we will dive into the topic of stress and how its control plays an essential role in kidney function. Imagine stress as a storm that, if not managed properly, can affect the serenity of your kidneys. We will explore in a clear and simple way why it is crucial to find ways to balance life and how to do it to strengthen your kidneys.

**A) How Stress Impacts the Kidneys**

Chronic stress can have negative effects on kidney health. When we experience stress, our body releases stress hormones, such as cortisol and adrenaline. These hormones, in excess, can contribute to problems such as high blood pressure, a risk factor for chronic kidney disease.

Additionally, stress can lead to unhealthy behaviors, such as overconsumption of unhealthy foods, lack of exercise, and poor quality sleep, all of which can negatively impact kidney health.

**B) The Stress-Kidney Disease Cycle**

Stress and kidney disease are often intertwined in a cycle. Kidney disease can increase stress due to health concerns, dietary restrictions, and the need for treatments. In turn, chronic stress can worsen kidney disease by contributing to hypertension and inflammation, factors that negatively affect the kidneys.

## C) Strategies to Control Stress

Now that we understand how stress can affect the kidneys, let's explore practical strategies to manage it and promote kidney peace.

- Relaxation Practices:
    - Incorporate relaxation practices such as meditation, deep breathing, or yoga into your daily routine. These techniques can reduce cortisol levels and promote calm.

- Time for Yourself:
    - Make time for activities that you enjoy and relax you. Whether reading, listening to music, taking a quiet walk or enjoying a relaxing bath, it is essential to reserve quiet moments.

- Regular Exercise:
    - Exercise is not only beneficial for physical health, but also for mental well-being. Physical activity releases endorphins, known as the "happiness hormones," which help combat stress.

- Organization and Planning:
    - Organize your time effectively and set realistic goals. The feeling of having control over your life and your responsibilities can reduce stress.

- Social support:
    - Share your worries with close friends or family. Social support is essential for coping with stress and can provide valuable perspective.

## D) Positive Impact on Kidney Health

Managing stress not only benefits mental health, but also has a positive impact on kidney health. By reducing the release of stress hormones and taking a more balanced approach to life, you can help keep your blood pressure within healthy limits and reduce the burden on your kidneys.

**E) Healthy Lifestyle as a Defense against Stress**

Adopting a healthy lifestyle is a powerful defense against chronic stress and its effects on kidney function. A balanced diet, regular exercise, and healthy sleep habits work together to strengthen not only your mental well-being, but also the health of your kidneys.

Conclusion: Balance for Stronger Kidneys

In short, stress control is like a balm for your kidneys, providing them with a calm environment conducive to their optimal functioning. By implementing strategies to manage stress, you can significantly contribute to kidney and overall health.

# 6.3 Tips for Restful Sleep and its Relationship with Kidney Health

**1. Sleep and Kidney Regeneration**

During sleep, your body carries out repair and regeneration processes, and your kidneys are no exception. Sleep quality is directly related to your kidneys' ability to perform their essential functions, such as filtering waste and maintaining fluid and electrolyte balance.

**2. Impact of Inadequate Sleep on Kidney Health:**

Lack of sleep or poor quality sleep can have negative consequences for kidney health. Studies have suggested that chronic sleep deprivation may contribute to the development of chronic kidney disease and increase the risk of hypertension, a risk factor for kidney problems.

**3. Establish a Sleep Routine**

Try to go to bed and wake up at the same time every day, even on weekends. This helps regulate your biological clock and improves sleep consistency.

**4. Create a Conducive Environment for Sleep**

Make sure your bedroom is dark, quiet and cool. Use blackout curtains, earplugs, or a white noise machine if necessary.

**5. Limit Screen Exposure Before Sleep**

Reduce time in front of electronic screens before bed. The blue light from these devices can interfere with the production of melatonin, the sleep hormone.

**6. Avoid Stimulants Before Sleep**

Limit caffeine consumption and avoid stimulating foods or drinks before bed. These can interfere with the quality of sleep.

**7. Do Physical Activity Regularly**

Regular physical activity can improve sleep quality. Try to exercise during the day, but avoid intense workouts right before bed.

**8. Establish a Relaxing Routine before Sleep**

Develop a relaxing bedtime routine, such as reading a book, taking a hot bath, or practicing meditation. These activities can help prepare your mind and body for sleep.

**9. Connection between Sleep and Blood Pressure**

Maintaining healthy blood pressure is crucial for kidney health, and sleep plays a significant role in this. During deep sleep, blood pressure decreases, allowing the cardiovascular system to relax and repair itself. Lack of sleep can contribute to hypertension, a risk factor for kidney problems.

**10. Melatonin and its Positive Impact**

Melatonin, the sleep hormone, not only regulates the sleep-wake cycle, but also has antioxidant and anti-inflammatory properties. These effects can help protect the kidneys against oxidative stress and inflammation, promoting their long-term health.

Restful sleep is like an elixir for your kidneys, providing them with the rest they need to function optimally. By adopting healthy sleep habits, you are investing in your body's kidney and overall health.

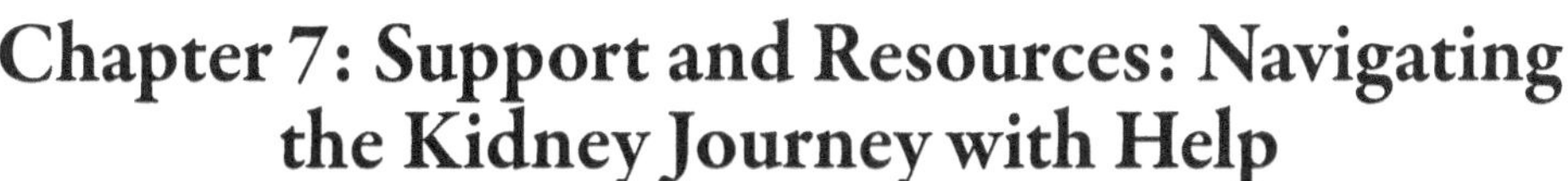

# Chapter 7: Support and Resources: Navigating the Kidney Journey with Help

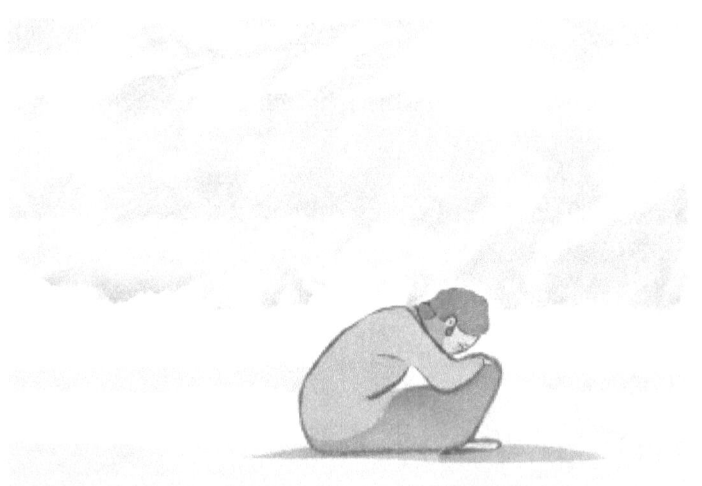

In this crucial segment of our kidney health journey, we will delve into the importance of support networks: family, friends, and support groups that can become critical pillars as we navigate the challenges and triumphs of maintaining healthy kidneys. . Visualize these networks as supportive arms that support you and accompany you every step of your journey.

## 7.1 Support Networks: Family, Friends and Support Groups

### Family: Unbreakable Pillars

Your family is like the anchor that keeps you steady through the waters of your kidney journey. They can be your parents, siblings, children, or anyone who shares close ties with you. Their emotional support, understanding, and active participation in your kidney care are invaluable.

- Open Communication:
    - Foster an environment of open communication with your family. Explain your situation, your needs and how they can support you. Mutual understanding will strengthen family ties and make facing challenges more bearable.

- Participation in Daily Care:
    - Invite your family to be part of your daily kidney care routine. Whether it's accompanying you to doctor's appointments, helping you prepare healthy meals, or simply providing company, their participation can ease the burden and create a sense of unity.

## Friends: Renal Travel Companions

Friends are like beacons that illuminate your path on your renal journey. They may be lifelong companions or new friends you meet in support groups or in the kidney community. Their emotional support and ability to share similar experiences can be a comforting balm.

- Meaningful Conversations:
    - Open meaningful conversations with your friends about your kidney health. Sharing your challenges and triumphs not only strengthens your friendship, but also raises awareness about the importance of kidney health.

- Celebrations and Shared Challenges:
    - Celebrate positive moments with your friends and seek support when you face challenges. Knowing that you are not alone in your kidney journey can make a difference in your outlook.

## Support Groups: Solidarity Communities

Support groups are like oases of understanding and compassion in the midst of the kidney journey. These groups bring together people who share similar experiences, providing a safe space for information exchange and emotional support.

- Active participation:
    - Join online or in-person support groups. Active participation will connect you with people who have been through similar situations and who can offer valuable advice and support.

- Continuous learning:
    - Take the opportunity to learn from the experiences of others in support groups. Questions about treatments, coping strategies and practical advice can enrich your own knowledge.

## How to Build and Strengthen your Support Networks

- Clear Communication:
    - Clear and honest communication is essential in all relationships. Express your needs, fears, and triumphs so your loved ones can better understand your situation.

- Kidney Health Education:
    - Provide information about kidney health to your loved ones so they better understand the challenges you face. Education can debunk myths and build a solid base of support.

- Celebrating Small Accomplishments:
    - Celebrate achievements, even the smallest ones. This not only boosts your own confidence, but also allows your loved ones to share in your joy and feel a part of your success.

- Search Online Resources:
    - Explore online resources, such as patient forums or social networks specializing in kidney health. These places can offer valuable connections and advice from people who are experiencing similar situations.

Support networks are like solid foundations that support your kidney journey. Your family, friends, and fellow support group members form a unique community that can make a difference in your well-being.

# 7.2 Role of the Medical Team in the Comprehensive Management of Kidney Disease

The medical teams are expert guides who accompany you, providing care, knowledge and support throughout your journey. Below we'll explain why having a strong medical team is essential and how working collaboratively with these professionals can strengthen your approach to optimal kidney health.

### A) The Medical Team as a Partner in Kidney Health

Your medical team is a group of health professionals who collaborate to provide you with the best possible care. This team may include nephrologists (kidney doctors), nurses, dieticians, social workers, and other specialists depending on your specific needs.

- Care Coordination:
  - The medical team is responsible for coordinating your comprehensive care. They work together to develop a personalized care plan that addresses all aspects of your kidney health, from medical treatment to emotional support.

- Continuous monitoring:
  - Your health professionals continually monitor your kidney health status. This involves regular blood tests, evaluations of kidney function, and adjustments to the treatment plan as necessary.

### B) Nephrologist: the Kidney Expert

A nephrologist is a doctor who specializes in kidney diseases and plays a central role in your medical team.

- Diagnosis and treatment:
  - The nephrologist evaluates your symptoms, performs diagnostic tests, and develops a treatment plan specific to your kidney condition. This may include medications, dietary changes, and other interventions.

- Long Term Monitoring:

- ○ Work with you to monitor your kidney health over the long term and adjust treatment as needed. Open communication with your nephrologist is essential for effective management.

## C) Nurses: Direct Support in Daily Care

Nurses play a crucial role in providing direct support and education about kidney care.

- Education and Counseling:
    - ○ Nurses educate you about administering medications, monitoring symptoms, and managing specific situations related to kidney disease. Their experience contributes to your ability to manage your kidney health in daily life.

- Link between Patient and Doctor:
    - ○ They act as an important link between you and your nephrologist. They report any changes in your condition to the medical team and provide you with the necessary care and support.

## D) Dietitian: Taking care of your Kidney Nutrition

The dietitian is a key member of the medical team, especially in the management of kidney diseases.

- Specific Diet Planning:
    - ○ Work with you to plan a specific diet that supports your kidney health. This involves controlling the intake of sodium, protein and other nutrients to avoid additional burden on the kidneys.

- Nutritional education:
    - ○ Provides personalized nutritional education so you can make informed decisions about your dietary choices. This is essential to control the progression of kidney disease and maintain overall health.

## E) Social Assistants: Emotional and Logistical Support

Caseworkers provide emotional support and help with logistics related to your kidney disease.

- Emotional Support:
    - They help manage the emotional impact of kidney disease, offering support and resources to deal with the stress, anxiety or depression that may arise.

- Resource management:
    - They assist with logistical issues such as coordinating insurance, obtaining financial resources, and advising on available support programs.

### F) Collaborative Work: Key to Success

Success in managing kidney disease lies in working collaboratively with your medical team.

- Open Communication:
    - Maintain open and honest communication with all members of your medical team. Share any symptoms, concerns or questions you may have.

- Active participation:
    - Actively participate in your kidney care. Understand your treatment plan, follow your medical team's recommendations, and ask questions when something is unclear.

Your medical team is a set of partners committed to your kidney journey. From the nephrologist to nurses, dieticians and social workers, each member plays a crucial role in your comprehensive care.

# 7.3 Online Resources and Kidney Patient Organizations

## Online Resources: A Virtual Library for Kidney Health

Online resources are like a virtual library that houses essential information on kidney health, treatments, lifestyle tips, and more. Accessing these resources empowers you with knowledge that will help you better understand your condition and make informed decisions.

- Trusted Websites:
    - Explore trusted websites that focus on kidney health, such as those provided by medical organizations, hospitals, or nephrology institutions. These sites usually offer accurate and up-to-date information.

- Online Forums and Communities:
    - Join online forums and communities focused on kidney health. These spaces allow you to connect with people who share similar experiences, ask questions, and receive emotional support from a supportive community.

- Educational Videos:
    - Take advantage of educational videos available on platforms like YouTube. Many healthcare organizations and professionals share valuable content that addresses specific topics related to kidney disease.

## **Kidney Patient Organizations: Companions on the Journey**

Kidney patient organizations are like expert companions on your kidney journey. These organizations are dedicated to providing support, education, and resources for those facing kidney challenges.

- Personalized Information:
    - These organizations offer personalized information about kidney disease, treatments, and strategies for daily management. You can trust that the information they provide is accurate and research-based.

- Events and Conferences:
    - Many kidney patient organizations organize events, conferences and webinars . These events are excellent opportunities to learn from experts, connect with other

patients, and get up-to-date information on advances in the field.

- Emotional Support Programs:
    - Some organizations offer emotional support programs, which may include helplines , in-person or online support groups, and resources to manage stress and anxiety related to kidney disease.

## How to Take Advantage of Online Resources and Kidney Patient Organizations

- Informed Research:
    - Do informed research using trusted online resources. Understanding the medical aspects of kidney disease allows you to make more informed decisions about your care and lifestyle.

- Active participation:
    - Actively participate in online communities and events organized by kidney patient associations. Share your experiences, ask questions and learn from others. Active participation strengthens your connection with the kidney community.

- Registration in Support Programs:
    - If an organization offers emotional support programs, sign up and participate. These programs can give you the support you need to cope with the emotional impact of kidney disease.

## Benefits of Connecting with Online Resources and Kidney Patient Organizations

- Emotional Support:
    - Connecting with other kidney patients through forums and support groups provides emotional support. Sharing your experiences and hearing those of others creates a sense of

community and understanding.

- Updated information:
    - Stay up to date with the latest information on treatments, research and advances in kidney health. Online resources and patient organizations are often reliable sources of up-to-date information.

- Personal Empowerment:
    - Accessing online resources and connecting with kidney patient organizations empowers you to be an effective advocate for your own health. The information and support you get helps you make informed and positive decisions.

Online resources and kidney patient organizations are like expert guides in kidney cyberspace. They offer you information, emotional support and valuable connections with a community that understands your challenges.

# Conclusion

As we come to the end of our book on kidney health, it is the perfect time to reflect on the valuable journey we have shared. Together, we have explored the fascinating world of our kidneys, essential organs that play a key role in keeping our body in balance. Throughout these pages, we have explored how to care for our kidneys, face challenges, and promote a full, healthy life.

Let's start by celebrating the wonder that is our kidneys. These organs work tirelessly behind the scenes, filtering waste and keeping our body in a state of balance. Although they often go unnoticed, our kidneys deserve our attention and care.

We have learned that prevention is key in kidney care. Adopting healthy daily habits, from a balanced diet to staying hydrated, is like giving our kidneys a daily hug. Every conscious choice is an investment in our long-term kidney health.

We've also explored the special bond between body and mind in the context of kidney health. We now understand that stress and emotional health can directly affect our kidneys. Taking care of our mental health is as important as taking care of our kidneys physically.

Throughout these pages, we have highlighted the strength that comes from connection with others. Whether through friends, family, online communities, or medical teams, mutual support creates a nurturing environment. Knowing that we are not alone in our kidney journey is a comforting reminder.

Continuing education has been a guiding light on our journey. Understanding how our choices affect our kidneys allows us to be active architects of our kidney health. Adaptability has also been a recurring theme, reminding us that life is full of change, and our approach to kidney health can evolve with us.

On our journey, we have celebrated every small achievement. Every step toward a healthier diet, every conscious lifestyle choice, and every day of kidney care are victories that deserve recognition. Celebrating these achievements propels us forward in a spirit of positivity and gratitude.

As we close this book, we realize that this is not an end, but a new beginning in our kidney journey. We look to the future with optimism and a renewed commitment to taking care of our kidneys. Kidney health is a continuous journey, and each day gives us the opportunity to strengthen our kidneys and improve our quality of life.

We want to express our sincere gratitude for joining us on this journey. Your dedication to kidney health and desire to learn and improve is inspiring. We hope this book has been more than words on paper; May it have been a practical and encouraging guide on your journey to stronger kidneys and a healthier life.

At this point in our journey, we invite you to continue exploring, learning, and applying what you have discovered. Every choice you make in your daily life is a step forward in your kidney journey. Let's continue the journey together , supporting each other and celebrating every milestone on our path to vibrant, long-lasting kidney health.

# Don't miss out!

Visit the website below and you can sign up to receive emails whenever Paul Sterling publishes a new book. There's no charge and no obligation.

https://books2read.com/r/B-A-OCJBB-YSESC

**BOOKS 2 READ**

Connecting independent readers to independent writers.

Did you love *Mastering Renal Health*? Then you should read *Managing Diabetes: Understanding and Controlling Type 1, Type 2, and Gestational Diabetes, Practical Strategies for Blood Sugar Management and Lifestyle Adaptation*[1] by Paul Sterling!

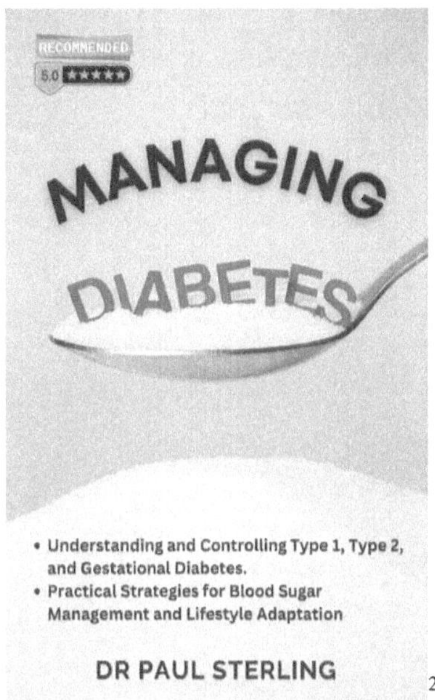


[2]

**<u>Are you ready to transform your relationship with diabetes?</u>**

**<u>"Managing Diabetes" is much more than a guide</u>**; It is your integral companion on the journey towards total control of your health. Written by experts in the field, this book unravels the mysteries of Type 1, Type 2, and Gestational Diabetes, providing you with practical strategies backed by the latest medical research.

<u>Imagine a future where diabetes no longer dictates your daily choices</u>, but you take control. From the moment you open the pages of this book, you will be immersed in a world of knowledge that will empower you to effectively manage your blood sugar and adapt to a lifestyle that promotes optimal health.

---

1. https://books2read.com/u/3RPajn

2. https://books2read.com/u/3RPajn

<u>**What can you expect from "Managing Diabetes"?**</u> From fundamental nutrition principles designed specifically for diabetic needs to tailored exercise strategies, each chapter is packed with practical tools to help you make informed decisions about your well-being.

Don't let diabetes be the narrator of your story; take the helm with "Controlling Diabetes." This book is your ticket to a future where you define the rules. Start your journey to freedom and lasting health today.

<u>**Your best version is waiting for you!**</u>

# Also by Paul Sterling

**Mejora tu Calidad de Vida**
Domina tu Salud Renal

**The Comprehensive Health Series**
Mastering Gastritis: Comprehensive Guide to Understanding and Treating Acute, Chronic, and Erosive Gastritis, plus Stomach Inflammation Management
Managing Diabetes: Understanding and Controlling Type 1, Type 2, and Gestational Diabetes, Practical Strategies for Blood Sugar Management and Lifestyle Adaptation
Mastering Renal Health

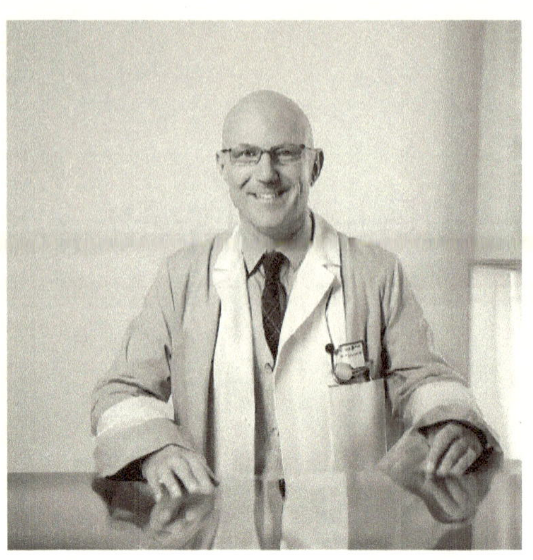

# About the Author

Dr. Paul Sterling is a respected medical researcher and prolific author, standing as an influential leader in the field of medicine. With a multifaceted career spanning various specialties, he has made an indelible mark on medical innovation. His passionate dedication to research and profound knowledge in diverse areas of medicine has positioned him as a trailblazer in the medical field. Recognized with numerous awards and honors, Dr. Sterling is distinguished by his unwavering commitment to improving healthcare and patient well-being. Additionally, as an accomplished author, he has written numerous acclaimed books that educate and inspire people of all ages on health topics. His ability to communicate complex medical concepts in an accessible manner makes him an exemplary educator, whose legacy will endure thanks to his tireless pursuit of excellence in medicine and his dedication to enhancing the lives of others.